CONTENTS

"What is to give light must endure burning."

-Viktor Frankl

"DIFFICULTIES STRENGTHEN THE MIND, AS LABOUR DOES THE BODY." - SENECA

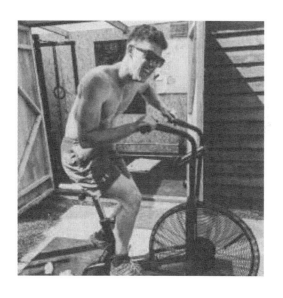

As fists pummelled into my teenage face, I knew what I should do: fight back, defend myself, or even run away. Yet I did nothing, and even when I squirmed so violently that I accidently kicked the other kid in the balls (giving me a second's opportunity for attack) I apologised profusely and allowed the beating to continue! To be fair, the punches and kicks stung. But the hardest blows were delivered by the rest of the school standing around cheering; my supposed friends included.

The rest of the day was spent feeling sorry for myself, sobbing. That was a typical day in my school life. I was scared and frightened. I was skinny, weak and lonely.

Now though, I can see that hardship was probably what made me who I am now. Those fragile years provided me with a lot of time to myself and the questions I had burned away in my mind. They started off as reflections of self-pity, but eventually morphed into various forms of the following:

- Why do we do the things we do?
- What makes someone successful?

- How do people make themselves do something they don't want to do?
- Why am I who I am?

But most important of all, the following question ate away at me:

> CAN I CHANGE THE PATH I'M ON? IS IT POSSIBLE FOR ME TO BE THE PERSON I WANT TO BE?

The answer, is *yes*.

That question took me places that I would never have believed possible: racking up over 10,000 hours of CrossFit coaching, becoming a Royal Marines Commando, developing a whole new level of confidence, forming a #1 ranked iTunes podcast, and also, what formed the subject of this book:

Creating a systematic approach for building the foundation of any athletic pursuit: Mindset RX'd.

The full Mindset RX'd system addresses all the difficulties an athlete[1] will experience: wanting to push harder, needing direction in their training (no goals/visions), creating a calm and quiet mind, visualising a workout effectively, and much more. But for now, as I'm sure you've realised from the title of the book, I'll be taking you through the process of developing consistency.

---

[1] An athlete is anyone on the path to becoming physically more able.

I used to waste a lot of time reading ineffectively; skimming over whole passages without absorbing anything; getting bored and distracted. I've discovered this method works well for me, so it may be a good place for you to start.

That being said, as with everything the principles are what matter. So please experiment and find what works for you.

I've also deliberately kept this book short. I could have written hundreds of thousands of words on this topic, but you don't get fitter/stronger/leaner/more mobile, by reading. So read, internalise, *then* apply it.

1. Use your finger or a pen and trace it along the words. This takes some getting used to (if you don't already do it) but

will slow you down a touch and keep your eyes focused on the section in view

2. Highlight important points or phrases.

3. Minimise distraction – I like to stick some headphones in (so people can see I won't be distracted). I'll listen to music without lyrics, specifically binaural beats.

4. Use the blank pages at the end of each chapter to summarise your thoughts.

WHY CONSISTENCY?

> **"WE ARE WHAT WE
> REPEATEDLY DO.**
> EXCELLENCE IS NOT AN ACT,
> BUT A HABIT." - ARISTOTLE

Just one thing separates you from your athletic potential. It's simple to understand, but hard to execute. The path to "success" is actually incredibly simple:

Do what works, consistently.

Learning what works, seems to have been the focus of training since training was first "a thing" in ancient Greece, almost 3,000 years ago. In this "information age", finding out what works is easy. In fact, it can be overwhelming when you start to see just how much information is available.

So, all that remains is to find a plan (follow programming at your box, eat paleo-ish and regular mobility work), then "just do it", right?

Wrong.

If only it were that simple. How many times have you started, then fallen off the wagon? How many times have you bought an Olympic weightlifting program, a membership to a mobility-based website, a new nutrition plan, then never started? How many new-year-new-me's have you experienced?

Finding answers is easy. Executing it however, is a whole new ball game.

When I was training for any single one of my goals, it was easy to find information, but no matter how perfect the plan, no matter how much thought I put into it, no matter how much I wanted it... I just couldn't *make* myself do it.

I would stick to the program for a few days, or if I was lucky, a few weeks. Then something would happen and I'd lose track again. Time and time again this would happen – for probably 3 years. Then, I was directed, as if by fate, to a book called *Bounce* by Matthew Syed. Now, having read it again, I can say the information in there is freely available, yet it triggered a realisation in me:

I AM FREE TO MAKE MY OWN DECISIONS.

I took ownership of the situation and threw myself into learning the questions I mentioned a few days back.

Over the years, I've tried countless methods to become more consistent. Some have worked, some haven't. What occurred to me, but was succinctly said by Gabe Rangel (hard-core to the extreme military member and awesome coach) on The Alpha Movement Podcast is this:

METHODS ARE MANY,
PRINCIPLES ARE FEW.

The following principles are what I've discovered:

1. Know yourself
2. Create a vision of success
3. Make it easy

So those are what we will be covering. Plus a bit more of course.

THE SUCCESS STRUCTURE

When most people think of the pillars of success, they usually think of something like the first image below.

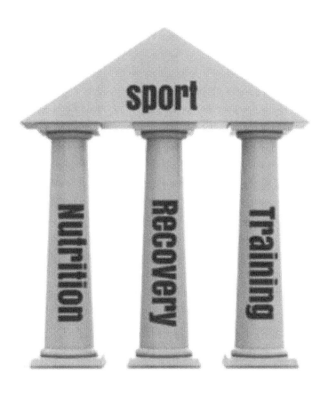

Which is great. The basic idea is this: you cannot build towards your goals if your nutrition training and recovery aren't in check. The training would include everything you do in the box, from your programming to your movement quality and everything in between.

Recovery is your soft tissue work, de-stressing, mindfulness practise, recovery runs etc. Nutrition is everything you put in your body.

But if you can't build towards your goals without having your nutrition, recovery and training in check, then it stands to reason that you can't build on any of these without first having your mindset in check.

Your mindset is the thing that allows you to do these things in the first place. It's the thing that allows you to do them consistently. It's what build your ability to success.

The model therefore, should look more like the image below:

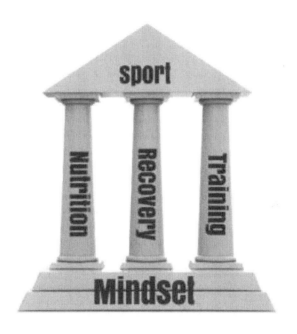

It's where you begin. Mindset is the Archimedes Lever that can both facilitate success and prevent it. It is the critical piece to your success as an athlete.

Master your mindset and you will leap forwards in your athletic potential.

Think back to the last time you started something and didn't finish it. Maybe a squat cycle? Hitting your macros? Gymnastics strength? Mobility?

Did you make it into a habit? Was it easy for you to do? Did you *want* to do it?

No, but you knew you should be doing it. And that is what mindset does; it lays a concrete foundation from which to create success.

By giving you a fail-proof system, we will show you exactly how to start enjoying your training again, be consistent, work harder than ever and therefore get stronger, fitter and healthier than ever before.

"YOU'VE JUST GOT TO WANT IT MORE"

How many times have you heard that phrase?

My opinion: it's bullshit.

If you think that works, consider this: do you think the overweight man who can't stick to a diet enjoys his knees hurting on every step? Do you think he doesn't want to blend in and avoid the judging looks? He desperately wants to change that, but he doesn't believe change is possible for him.

If you've been told in the past "you've just got to want it more", then it's spurred you into action for a couple of weeks, that's because of *guilt* or *fear*. I don't know about you, but I don't want either of those two to be my motivating factors!

There's a myriad of techniques in the mainstream like this that just don't fucking work! I want to show you the truth. That's why I've written this book.

CHAPTER 1: THE COMPETENCE SPECTRUM

When you begin a new routine, it's easy to you. The novelty of the process and excitement of the end goal make the first portion of any new activity or habit easy.

With excitement and relish, we smash the first few days. We tell our friends how well we're doing. We can see the progress you're making and the end goal seems closer already.

Then, for some reason, you wake up one morning and don't feel like doing it. Maybe something has popped up in your personal life. So you miss "just this one day" and promise you'll be back on it tomorrow. Needless to say, a few weeks later, you're not performing the habit you once loved doing.

At this point, you're likely to move onto the next goal. Hold on though, because you're actually over a quarter of the way to making this a permanent habit. In fact you're at stage 1 of 4.

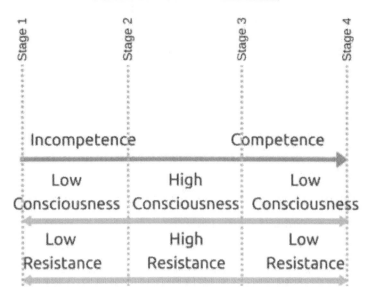

THE COMPETENCE SPECTRUM

Before I identify the stages, let me define some terms.

Competence: Performing a behaviour that serves you/that you want to perform (a beneficial behaviour)

Incompetence: Not doing said behaviour

Consciousness: How much you have to think about performing the behaviour

Resistance: How difficult it is to perform the beneficial behaviour

So, as you progress from incompetence to competence, you can see that both the resistance and the consciousness increase. As it becomes habitual though, the consciousness required and the resistance both diminish.

Along the way to competence, you will hit 4 stages:

1. Unconscious incompetence
2. Conscious incompetence
3. Conscious competence
4. Unconscious competence

Picture this:

You're driving along in the car, someone cuts you up. Without thinking, you slam your fist on the horn and shout at them (unconscious incompetence). But I'm in the car and I look pretty pissed off with your lack of self-control so you think *actually, maybe that wasn't cool...I'd like to change that behaviour*.

So a few days pass before almost exactly the same thing happens. You again slam your fist down on the horn and shout. But this time, there's a fraction of a second when you realise what you're about to do... but you do it anyway! Of course, you're at conscious incompetence.

A few days after that, the same thing happens and it requires every ounce of self-control, tongue biting and restraint to let it go. Well done, you're now at conscious competence. Repeat this enough, and eventually you'll perform the behaviour without thought – unconscious competence.

Does it always happen this smoothly? No. Are there slight deviations depending on the person and the habit? Of course. But we do know that everyone pretty much follows this path, as long as they keep taking steps forwards.

So, next time when you find it difficult to prep your meals or do your mobility/accessory work know this: you've just reached a milestone along the way. You've just made progress. Let's take another step.

But that's enough of the theory. Let's get into the actual steps on becoming more consistent.

CHAPTER 2: AN INTRODUCTION TO THE PYRAMID

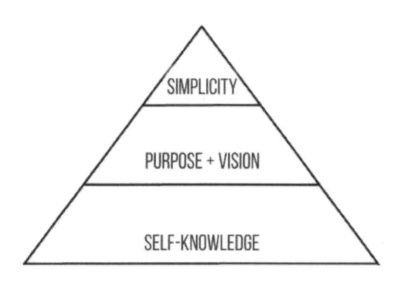

Years of work, trial and error, and research have produced this pyramid. I've watched countless people succeed in becoming more consistent and even more fail in the quest. I was puzzled as to why people some people managed it with ease and some people didn't, despite trying to do the same thing with almost similar outside demands.

Having now used this new format with dozens if not hundreds of athletes, I am happy to say, this is the most effective version yet.

If you've read *Start With Why* by Simon Sinek, you may recognise part of this. Essentially, the *what* is the last thing we'll touch upon. The *how* and the *why* are in the middle. But we'll add another layer which forms the foundation: *who* which takes the form of self-knowledge.

CHAPTER 3: SELF-KNOWLEDGE

"YOU HAVE POWER OVER YOUR MIND – NOT OUTSIDE EVENTS. REALIZE THIS, AND YOU WILL FIND STRENGTH." –
MARCUS AURELIUS

Knowing yourself: what drives you, what is an energy sap for you, what makes you happy, what you find easy and all the rest of it, is what people most often forget. Coaches are often quick to provide a method, but reluctant to make sure you do it.

Which is why we start with *who*.

The second part of the self-knowledge thought process, is the idea that one-size-fits-one. At the end of this book, I'm going to give you a few tools to get started. But it's important to remember, you are you. Only you have had your exact experiences, so test and retest. See what works.

For now though, spend some time asking the following questions.

- What has driven you in the past?

....
....
....
....
....
....
....

- What's your biggest success?

....
....
....
....
....
....
....

- Who do you want to be for your family?

....
....
....
....
....
....
....

- Who do you want to be for yourself?

....
....
....
....
....
....
....

- What makes you happy?

....
....
....

....
....
....
....

- When was the last time you felt fearless?

....
....
....
....
....
....

Most of all...

- *Who do you want to be?* Not what do you
  want to achieve. Not how are you going
  to do it or why. *Who* is the person you'd
  love to see looking back at you in the
  mirror?

....
....
....
....

....
....
....
....
....
....
....
....

"THE SECRET OF CHANGE IS
TO FOCUS ALL YOUR ENERGY
NOT ON FIGHTING THE OLD,
BUT ON BUILDING THE NEW." -
SOCRATES

Once you have a deeper understanding of your true motivations, we can create vision of what you'd like to achieve. This vision is what we'll come back to when times are tough.

Please note, having a vision is very different from having goals. Goals are merely mile markers on the highway to our vision. A vision is a full sensory experience of our desired outcome – the emotions, the sight, the sound, the feel and even the smell and taste.

The reason we create a vision of success, is because the human brain is an extremely powerful tool we have at our disposal. In fact, it's incredibly poor at telling "reality" from our imagination – trust me on this, there's a multitude of studies proving this. In fact, if you repeat a thought often enough in your mind, you'll not only start to believe it, but begin to act like it's true.

That's why the best athletes can appear a touch arrogant – it's simply that they believe they are the best in the world. Because of this, they begin acting like it. When they begin acting like it, they start achieving the things the best in the world is likely to achieve. Because they achieve it, the belief is reinforced.

The opposite is true too. Ever met one of those people who tells you how they're always unlucky? Yeah the bad luck follows them around, right? It's not a coincidence.

Your beliefs are your life.

So, what we do, is we use our knowledge of ourselves to tap into what means a lot to us. From that, we can create a vision of success in our minds. Don't skimp on this; it's powerful shit!

We then repeat it on a daily basis – I like to write mine out.

Important: this is not an affirmation. Just because you say something, it doesn't mean it's magically going to happen. It does mean that you will see the opportunities around you and begin to unravel some of the stories about yourself that you think are true.

Use the following pages to scribble down some ideas:

"COMPLEXITY IS THE
ENEMY OF EXECUTION" –
TONY ROBBINS

We're often under the illusion that bigger is better. That more is preferable. More weight on the bar, more reps in the time domain, more chalk (okay maybe that one's true).

When it comes down to forming habits though, less really is more. The less we have to do, the more likely we are to do it. Let's attack a common downfall for people: nutrition.

You catch sight of yourself in a picture on social media from the box. You're not the focus of the picture, but you're in the background and it's like "jeeez.... when did I begin looking like that?" So, drastic action is taken. You decide that enough is enough, and this time...*this time*... I'm doing it right. You borrow the box's copy of The Zone Diet, calculate your blocks, then print off a perfect program after 6 hours of work. You're ready to rock and roll! Let's do this!

The reality is, you haven't even started. You've still got to buy the food, weigh the food, spend a whole Sunday batch cooking it, buy the Tupperware because the lids have all gone missing, freeze some, order your supplements, buy a new shaker, wash it up every night, and you haven't even got to the first day yet!

So, consider that option 1.

Option 2 takes a slightly different approach:

Week 1: begin tracking what you eat and when (not calculating macros)

Week 2: remove white carbs + excess sugar

Week 3: make sure you're getting 2.5l of water a day

Week 4: Calculate your macros and begin to stick within 10% either side

Etc.

What sounds more achievable?

I know which approach I'd rather stick to.

The same is true with mobility. You want an all singing, all dancing 21 day revolving program? Well, how about you commit to just 30 seconds a day to begin with. This is the thing to consider: In the initial stages, getting the benefit from the activity isn't the most important outcome, setting up a habit that works is.

That there, is the most important aspect of the simplicity segment.

When it comes to choosing the first activity, I find this question always comes in handy.

"If I could only do one thing, what would I do?" or to get further into it, "what one activity, if done well, will render the others obsolete?" If you don't know the answer, ask someone who does.

In the nutrition example above, I always begin with just tracking with most people, especially beginners. This is because it brings about a higher level of consciousness regarding food choices. When I was still working with athletes on their nutrition, I would get great results from only getting them to track their food intake. They would make better choices as a result of that.

Regardless of where an athlete fits into my Mindset Models (as I mentioned earlier, I don't have the space in this small book to go into them in much detail) they all start with these 2 activities, performed on a daily basis.

JOURNALING

Journaling is how we learn to tap into our subconscious. This is how we discover what is limiting us as athletes. Now, I get what journaling sounds like to you: "dear diary…". It's not writing a letter to an imaginary being, it's just allowing your thoughts to be heard consciously.

So, every morning grab a pen and paper and let your thoughts come out on the paper. It sometimes helps to prompt your mind by thinking about training.

Do not filter. Do not edit. Listen and write. Do not judge but dictate your subconscious thoughts on to the page.

Beware of being misled by the simplicity of this exercise or even any judgements about it. It is powerful in guiding you to being a better athlete and fulfilling your potential. We are just doing this for a fixed term – 7-10 days – and it's just 2-5 minutes at a time.

What we do from that point, is skim for consistent thought patterns, then we can act...The process after that, is completely dependent on the thoughts you're having.

This is an excellent way to tap further into your mind than you will do with the questions I asked in the "self-knowledge" chapter.

I could write thousands of words to try and convey how powerful this exercise is, but Frankie, one of my old personal training clients said it best: "I had no idea how fucking mean I was to myself". This hits the nail on the head. If someone else said the things you say to yourself, you'd knock them out!

Counting Wins

A lot of people lose the consistency battle because they fail to recognise just how far they're coming. Unfortunately, success isn't linear. It comes in floods, then we experience a success drought. In need of an exercise that keeps us positive, I borrowed/adapted/stole an exercise from the guys I consider my mentors in this space.

It's simple in concept and elegant in execution. All you do, is write down every single thing you've done that day which you consider a win. They can be training related, or they can be from the rest of your life. Nothing is irrelevant or stupid. If something made you happy, stick it in there.

If you're ever feeling a bit bleurgh, have a flick through too. You'll realise how much closer you are to achieving your target.

If you ever feel like not counting your wins, then this is a sure-fire sign that you must!

Take this quote from Dan, an athlete I'm working with right now: "I never knew how much I was doing every day that was making me better. I guess you just get used to it and get frustrated..."

I know both of these activities may seem a touch simple to be really effective, but I assure you, there's great power in this.

Firstly, the journaling is a sure-fire way to discover beliefs that are limiting your progress. In fact, I've had people in the Inner Athlete Performance Camp who have just done this and changed their beliefs and achieve their athletic potential! Whilst this is rare, and most people need the full techniques on offer in the Inner Athlete Performance Camp, it does occasionally happen.

Win counting is great too despite, or rather because of, its simplicity. It takes just a few minutes and can take you from feeling like you've achieved nothing to realising that you're much closer to your objective despite not having the best of days. That's the difference between taking another step forwards tomorrow, and not. To put it another way, it's the difference between success and failure.

3 WAYS MASTERING YOUR INNER ATHLETE WILL TRIGGER A PR LANDSLIDE

Boxes are teeming with athletes who will do anything for a PR. The shortcut, the edge, the unknown secret. We mine Google and social media for nuggets, believing that the obstacle to overcome is a lack of information. If only it were that easy!

The real barrier to success lies in your mind. I call it your Inner Athlete. Let me explain:

Objectivism

When we haven't mastered our Inner Athlete, we rarely see a situation for what it really is; we tarnish it with the brush of that moment's mood. This can work in one of a few ways, depending on which mindset model you fall into.

Firstly, you could always be looking on the positive side of the equation. That niggle in your shoulder? That will be fiiiiiine. It always has been after all...

Or... just one extra cheat meal won't hurt... will it?

The opposite is of course true also.

You're just not improving... what's the point of trying.

You never have been good, you're not going to get any better.

Can't teach an old dog new tricks...

It's common for people to flip between the two as well. One moment, you feel on top of the world. The next, you're helpless.

When we master our Inner Athlete, we are given perspective on a situation. We see a situation for what it really is and because of that we can judge what the appropriate action to take is.

This alone, is one of the biggest differences between those who succeed in a physical challenge and those who don't.

Intensity Tolerance

At both the highest levels of the sport, and the grass roots, athletes who set PRs are all willing to tolerate intensity to a high level. Not only the discomfort of actually setting the PR, but the training to be facilitate it.

Most of us live in a bubble; air-conditioning, food on demand, sheltered sleeping all make the need of intensity tolerance largely unnecessary. We no longer require regular exposure to hardship in order to survive. This is undoubtedly a good thing. But the human mind is wired for survival. As such, given the opportunity, most of us will take the easier choice. I mean, why struggle?

Unfortunately, we don't rise to our expectations but sink to the level of our training. Therefore we must not only accept hardship to improve as an athlete, but embrace it.

When we have tamed you inner athlete, you will enjoy the process of getting uncomfortable. As a result, the training will yield better returns, the PR attempts will require less motivation and PRs will cascade.

Perpetual Positivity

Remember what it felt like last time you crushed a WOD? That unbeatable feeling... The sound... the experience... the exhaustion mixed with excitement...

Well, imagine how much you'd achieve if you felt even 10% of that on a daily basis. You wouldn't let the situation get you down. The soreness and fatigue would begin to become irrelevant. You'd be a man/woman on a mission!

That's what all the best athletes have and that's what I try to cultivate in the Inner Athlete Performance Camp. An athlete who has mastered their Inner Athlete understands the journey they are on. They feel good about the situation, whatever it throws at them because they know, whether it's good or bad, they are in control.

To master your Inner Athlete, you need to get specific to you; one size really does fit one. You need to find out which of the four mindset models you are currently operating from, plus you need to find out what your point B really is.

To say *thank you* for purchasing this book, I'd like to guide you through this process on a 1-2-1 basis. This will take the form of a 30 minute GRIT call with myself. Having given hundreds of these calls now, I'll ensure you finish the call with a great understanding of yourself and a plan to get where you want to be.

Essentially, this will be the call that facilitates you becoming the best version of yourself possible. It's the call that allows you to be better tomorrow than you are today. It's a shortcut that throws out trial and error and replaces it with direction and certainty.

I'm going to cut off the offer for GRIT calls at some point too. When that happens, I'll be cutting this final section from the book. So if you're reading this, you have a chance – act soon!

To hop on your GRIT call with me, just email tom@alphamovement.co with the subject "FREE GRIT CALL".

I'm really looking forward to showing you how to apply this to your life and achieving your vision as a result of that.

Best,

Tom

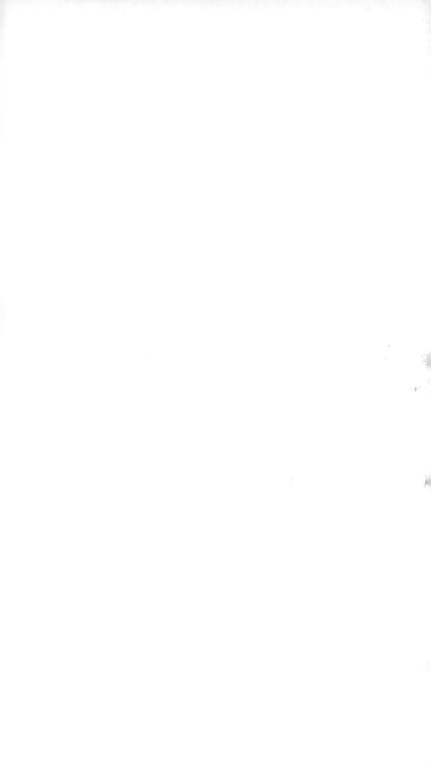

25247084R10031

Printed in Great Britain
by Amazon